THE
Jewish Baby
HANDBOOK

T0268433

PRESENTED TO

_____

BY

_____

DATE

_____

THE
Jewish Baby
HANDBOOK
A Guide for Expectant Parents

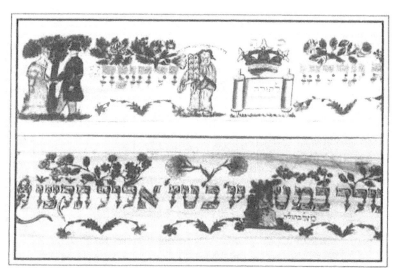

RABBI   DOUGLAS   WEBER
JESSICA   BRODSKY   WEBER

BEHRMAN HOUSE

DEDICATED TO OUR PARENTS
Jack and Adele Brodsky
Stan and Renee Weber

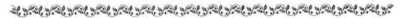

PROJECT EDITOR: RUBY G. STRAUSS

BOOK DESIGN: BARBARA HUNTLEY

COVER PHOTO: "FIRST STEPS"/VINCENT VAN GOGH
THE METROPOLITAN MUSEUM OF ART, GIFT OF
GEORGE N. AND HELEN M. RICHARD, 1964.
(64.165.2) PHOTOGRAPH BY MALCOLM VARON.

COPYRIGHT © 1990 BY BEHRMAN HOUSE, INC.

235 WATCHUNG AVENUE, WEST ORANGE, NJ 07052

ISBN-0-87441-499-7

MANUFACTURED IN THE UNITED STATES OF AMERICA

07 06 05 04

CONTENTS

"The mitzvah of being fruitful and multiplying exists so that the earth will be settled. And it is a great mitzvah . . . because of it, all the others exist."

SEFER HINNUKH, BREISHIT

You're expecting a baby—Mazal Tov!

NOTHING changes one's life as much as the experience of becoming a parent. The "before child" world of personal quiet time and freedom of movement is quickly replaced by the serious and seemingly endless responsibility of caring for a human being totally dependent on you for every need.

Before we had our kids, people tried to describe the experience to us, to let us know what to expect. We learned how to breathe through contractions, how to diaper and burp. We read books on fetal development and discussed the ways in which our relationship would become strained. But, despite the best efforts, we were not entirely prepared for what was to come, for a birth, and the creation of a new family unit, is an intensely emotional experience, one that can only be truly understood as it occurs. One thing is for certain. Life is never quite the same again.

Imagine for a moment a scene at the beach in summer. Children romp in the ocean and dig in the sand. Parents are unable to fully relax, for they have to make sure that their children don't eat sand, or drown in the waves. Anyone would long for the "pre-child" days, days of lying on a blanket, listening to the surf, and reading a book. Yet, it is the parents who are the lucky ones. They are the ones who experience the joys and pleasures of play, along with their children. They are the ones who have the opportunity to be children once more, to grow up all over again, to feel life's surprises as though they are new.

For Jewish parents, the experience goes even deeper, for just as we strive to perpetuate ourselves personally, we as a people have always been driven to perpetuate Torah. What is Torah without children to receive it? What is Judaism without the links of the generations? Our children not only bring us to life, they bring our Judaism to life.

So, on two counts we wish you a hearty *mazal tov*. For yourself, for you will have the wonderful opportunity to grow up all over again with someone new and beautiful to love, and for the Jewish people, whose love of God and Torah will continue for yet another generation.

We hope that this handbook will give you food for thought as the birth of your new baby draws near. We have tried to be mainstream in our presentation, but as we all know, for every Jew there are at least two opinions. Issues of Jewish law and denominationalism are not fully explored here, and in some areas there is a wider range of opinion and practice than what is presented. If you wish further information on any of these topics, or if you have additional questions, you should consult your rabbi.

With each new experience our Jewish knowledge grows. Often it is our children who force us closer to our faith. See . . . they're doing it even before they are born!

"There is no time a man spends on earth that he enjoys
more than the time he spends in the womb."

TALMUD BAVLI, NIDAH 30B

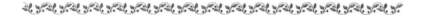

*What did our sages understand
about gestation?*

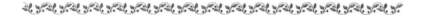

THE rabbis of the Talmud offer
us advice and information on a myriad of topics. Their advice,
was based on observation, on the spiritual and legal framework
of the tradition, and on the latest scientific data of their day.
One of these topics is gestation, and while the rabbis were
certainly not experts in the area, they showed great interest in
it, and devoted much space to it in the pages of the Talmud.
Their stories and thoughts on the subject are not to be taken in
the same way as information that we might glean from pre-natal
and birth classes. They do represent, however, a spiritual look
at our struggle to understand how life comes about. In this
sense, the rabbis offer us wisdom valid in any age.

One Talmudic midrash explains that there are three partners
in the creation of a child: the father, the mother, and God. The
father provides the white matter, such as the bones, sinews,
nails, brain and the whites of the eyes. The mother provides the
red matter which forms the flesh, the hair, the blood, the skin
and the dark of the eyes. God offers the spirit, the breath, the
beauty of the features, the ability to see, hear, think, speak and
walk.

Another midrash goes as follows:

At conception, God forces a soul to enter the new being. The soul is reluctant to do so, for it does not want to give up its freedom for a stay on earth. Yet, it has no choice. In utero, a light burns over the new child's head, enabling it to see from one end of the earth to the other. The child has complete knowledge of Torah, and has full understanding of life and death. Just before birth, the child is touched by an angel, causing her to forget this infinite wisdom. Folklore tells us that the indentation of the upper lip is the permanent sign of that angel's touch.

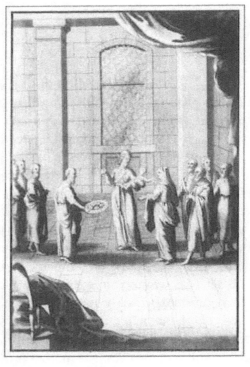

*Engraved depiction of Redemption
of the First-Born
18th century Holland*

"Legend always contains a grain of law."
RABBI ABRAHAM ISAAC KOOK, OROT HAKODESH

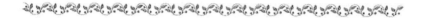

What folk customs surround the birth of a baby?

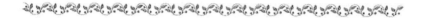

THE months before our first child was born were filled with excitement and expectation. We couldn't wait to buy the crib and the other necessary items for the new nursery. We went shopping and selected furniture, and a mobile (so the baby would be able to begin his intellectual development), and asked the proprietor of the store to deliver it all. He wouldn't do it. A Jewish man, the father of a friend, Lenny would not allow us to bring the baby items into our home before the baby was born. "Just in case something happens, God forbid," he told us, "You won't want all this stuff lying around. Call me the minute the baby is born and I'll have it all there in an hour!" We had no choice and went home empty handed.

Sure enough, when our son was born, Lenny had everything waiting for us when we came home from the hospital, just as he had said, with a bottle of shnaps thrown in for good luck.

The superstition (or *bubeh meiseh*) of not physically preparing one's home for a new baby, of not having a baby shower until after the baby is born, is really not so foolish. Even though the original intent had to do with demons and bad luck, the logic of not celebrating until there is something to celebrate is psychologically sound. We shouldn't be quick to dismiss folk belief, for sometimes there is wisdom at the core.

Folk customs surrounding birth are numerous in every culture. Jews have picked up these beliefs from our neighbors in various places around the world, and made them our own. Placing the circumcision knife under the pillow of the mother the night before the brit, to protect her from demons, follows similar customs in other cultures where weapons of iron are kept near newborns. Amulets to ward off evil spirits are used in many traditions, but Jewish amulets contain verses from the Psalms especially the verse, "The sun shall not smite thee by day, neither the moon by night." *(Psalm 21:6).*

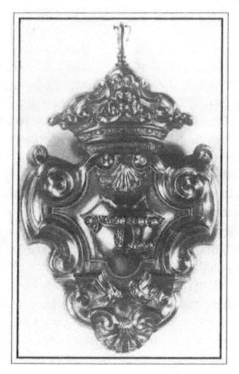

Gold Amulet
17th century Italy

There are many other folk customs, some of which you might know from your own family. Here are a few:

1. The custom of not announcing a child's name until the circumcision or naming ceremony comes from the Talmudic concept that the baby is not entirely viable until the eighth day.

2. Garlic and red ribbons were placed on the baby's crib to protect it from the evil eye, or demons. Lilith, one such demon, is specifically suspected of stealing small children for herself, since, as legend has it, she is forever bitter about her own inability to bear children.

3. Yemenite Jews place sweets under the bed of the new mother to occupy the evil spirits and to draw attention away from the baby.

4. During difficult labor, Ashkenazi Jews would sometimes put a Torah binder around the belly of the woman, or put the keys to the synagogue in her hands.

5. In ancient Israel, it was customary to plant a tree for the new baby.

A friend once confessed that she responded to any and all charity solicitations during her pregnancies. "That's the time when you really can't fool around," she said. Despite our sophisticated attitudes in terms of modern science and technology, to discard entirely our folk customs would be to assume that we have total control over our lives and our environment.

So, even if we don't want garlic on the crib, and even if we feel that candy under the bed will bring bugs, we can always give extra tzedakah. That never hurts!

"For this child I prayed . . ."

I SAMUEL 1:27

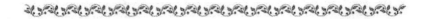

Is there a blessing to recite upon the birth of a baby?

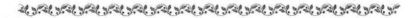

OUR tradition offers us a wide vocabulary of blessings. In reciting them, we acknowledge God's role in providing our food, our health, the beauties of nature, the Torah, our holidays, and for enabling us to reach landmark events in our lives. We have blessings to mark the small, simple moments, as well as the less frequent but special times—words of praise that turn these experiences into holy events. Blessings teach us to sanctify time and insure that we will not take anything for granted.

Most blessings begin with the same formula, "Baruch atah adonai eloheinu melech haolam . . . " (Blessed are you, the Eternal, our God, ruler of the universe . . .), and conclude with the appropriate phrase. Some are long, like the five paragraph blessing we recite after we read the haftarah, and some are simple, like the single sentence we say over wine.

It is odd, therefore, considering the importance we place on blessings within our tradition, that there is no specific blessing or ritual to mark the moment of birth. Perhaps, if the rabbis had been the ones actually giving birth, a customary blessing would have been recorded. Since none has, many women feel that it is time to create this new ritual.

Blu Greenberg, a well known voice among liberal Orthodox women, suggests that parents recite the same blessing that is used upon hearing any good news. It goes as follows: "Baruch atah adonai, eloheinu melech haolam, hatov vehameytiv." In English it reads, "Blessed are you, the Eternal, our God, ruler of the universe, who is good and does good."

The book *Gates Of Mitzvah*, published by the Reform movement, cites the Sheheheyanu blessing as one that is appropriate for that occasion. This blessing is said upon having any experience for the first time, and goes as follows: "Baruch atah adonai, eloheinu melech haolam, sheheheyanu, vekimanu, vehigianu lazman hazeh." In English it reads, "Blessed are you, the Eternal, our God, Ruler of the universe, who has given us life, sustained us, and helped us to reach this special day."

The following prayer of thanksgiving has been offered within the Reconstructionist movement: "How wonderful is this moment as we stand at the edge of the mystery of life. Our daughter/son, how small and beautiful you are . . . Let our arms be your love cradle; our whispered prayer, your lullaby song . . . In awe and gratitude for this precious gift of life, we celebrate our partnership in the miracle of creation."

It is certainly proper to offer a blessing of thanks at the completion of such a monumental event as a birth. By remembering to thank God, we give ourselves the opportunity to create special "kodesh" or a holy moment in our lives and to appreciate the grandeur of life.

"A fair name is better than precious balm."
ECCLESIASTES 7:1

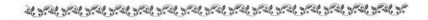

What should we name the baby?

CHOOSING names can be wonderful experience. To select for sound and tone, for historical significance and meaning, an aspect of human beings that they will carry with them all their lives is a creative opportunity. When we select a name, we think of what we wish that child to be like. We think of loved ones, no longer with us, whose examples we wish them to follow. We send our children out into the world with the best names we can offer, and hope that, as adults, they will like the ones we chose.

Jewish names come from several sources. Traditionally, the first source has always been the Bible. The names of the righteous, brave and generous personages in the Scriptures have always been popular. "Have you ever heard that a man should call his son Pharoah? Better Abraham, Isaac, Jacob, Reuben, Simon, Levi, or Judah." *(Gen. R49:1)*. As the Talmud tells us, the name of a person can determine his destiny. *(Ber. 7b)*.

A recent trend has been toward modern Hebrew names which include aspects of nature, as well as other picturesque nouns and verbs. These are used more frequenlty for girls, since the Bible is a much richer source of male names. Several Jewish name dictionaries offer many possibilities.

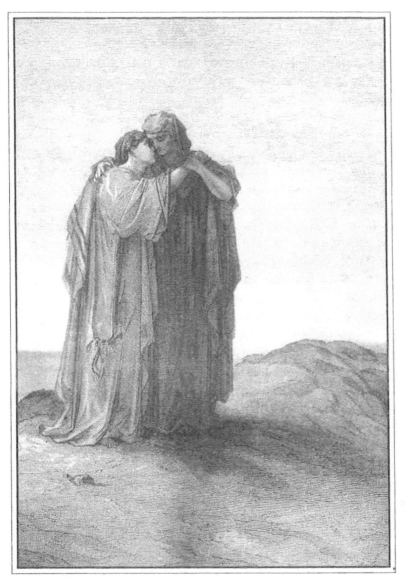

Naomi and her daughter-in-law Ruth
Paul Gustave Dore, 17th century England

A third source of Jewish names has always been the surrounding culture within which we live. Even the rabbis of the Talmud are sometimes recognized with Greek names such as Antigonus and Avtalyon. Some of our names are translations of Hebrew into a vernacular, such as Moses for Moshe, or Suzanne for Shoshannah. In any case, when using English names, or names in another foreign tongue, it is not traditional to choose ones with Christian connotation.

It has been a long standing custom in the Jewish community to have a civil name along with a Jewish name. It is convenient here to bridge the gap between the two by providing an English name with a Hebrew equivalent, such as David or Miriam. Names can also be paired by sound, as is Jason for Grandpa Jack or by meaning as is Bloomah, (meaning flower), for Great Grandma Florence, (also meaning flower).

In terms of our Hebrew names, we follow the ancient custom of calling ourselves by a first name, and then the son or daughter of our parents. For example, the biblical Jacob was called Yakov Ben Yitzhack, or Jacob the son of Isaac. Rachel was known as Rachel Bat Laban, or Rachel the daughter of Laban. Many modern Jews now include the mother's name as well, so that both parents are represented in the child's Hebrew name.

European Ashkenazic tradition discourages the naming of a child after someone who is living. In the Sephardic tradition, however, naming children after living persons is permissible and common, though these rarely include parents.

Formal Hebrew names are given at either the *brit milah* ceremony or at the naming ceremony. We are known by them within the Jewish community, using them when we are called to the Torah and during lifecycle events. When we are called to the Torah as a Bar/Bat Mitzvah, when we recite marriage vows under the huppah, when we are eulogized, it is by our Hebrew name that we are known.

It is interesting to note that Jews did not always have last names. Surnames were not necessary when Jews lived in small towns and had little contact with the outside world. Someone could have been called Chaim ben Moshe all his life, never needing a last name. Or he could have been called Chaim the Baker, based on his profession. About 200 years ago, European countries began requiring Jews to take last names and to officially register them.

Jews most often created their last names from their professions or from the names of their towns and cities. The name Weber is German for weaver, and the name Brodsky means "son of Brod", a Polish town. Some names came from personal characteristics such as Gross, Weiss and Schwartz. These names soon took root and were passed from generation to generation. They became the names that we now know as "Jewish" names, though we should keep in mind that in terms of Jewish history, they aren't very old at all.

> "Who circumcises his son is as though he offered
> all the sacrifices to the Lord."
>
> ZOHAR 95A

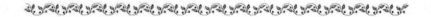

What is a brit milah?

BRIT, (bris in Yiddish) is the
Hebrew word for "covenant"; *milah* means "circumcision".
The Torah describes a series of covenants. The universal *brit*
between God and all humanity was made through Noah; the
great covenant at Sinai was made with the Jewish people in
particular. A critical step in this evolution is described in
Genesis 17, where God commands Abraham to bear the mark
of his special relationship to God in his (and his descendents')
flesh.

Shrouded in pre-history, the act of removing the foreskin
which covers the glans of the penis certainly existed before
Abraham's time. It was practiced by a variety of ancient cultures
before being invested with the overtly religious significance it
took on in Judaism. Philo of Alexandria, (living in Hellenistic
culture and seeking to demonstrate the compatibility of Torah
and reason), described *milah* as a method to safeguard
cleanliness and health. Maimonides, (who similarly made great
efforts to harmonize Torah with the science of his day), viewed
circumcision as a means to curb lust, and as a symbol of
sacrifice.

The importance of *milah* to Jewish survival has always been perceived by anti-Semites. The familiar Hanukkah story begins in 165 B.C.E. with a royal decree forbidding circumcision in an attempt to destroy Jewish distinctiveness. Three centuries later, the Hadrianic persecutions focused on what Rome saw as the cornerstones of Jewish identity: study of Torah and the practice of *brit milah*. Over the millenia, Jews and their detractors have agreed on this point: without *brit milah*, the Jews as a people would not last long.

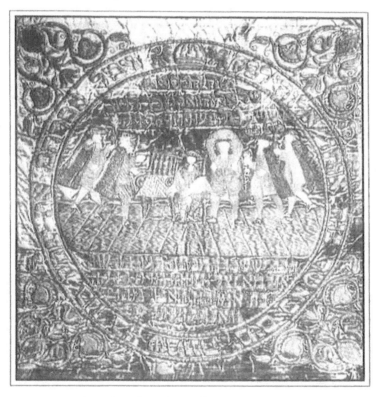

*Embroidered Cushion for Circumcision Bench
Germany, 1729*

Under normal circumstances, infant boys undergo the minor operation. Bleeding is usually very limited. Detailed and exact instructions on the dressing and care of the minor wound are given. Usually a complete healing takes place in just a few days. In our experience, the psychological trauma felt by the parents of the newborn far exceeds the physical discomfort of the baby.

Debate continues and surely always shall, over the medical necessity or advisability of routine circumcision. Advocates of the procedure point to statistically lower rates of cervical cancer and pelvic inflamatory disease among women whose sexual partners are circumcised. Detractors see the operation—from a strictly medical perspective—as superfluous in an age of better hygienic conditions.

These developments highlight the essential *religious* nature of *brit milah*. Like many *mitzvot* (e.g. *kashrut*) there may be health advantages, or (like *Shabbat*) good common sense benefits. These however, remain secondary to the purpose of *mitzvot* which is to draw us closer to God and increase a sense of *kedushah* (sanctity) in our lives.

The true sense of *brit milah* is only understood fully when the words are joined together. All humankind enjoys a *brit* ("covenant") with God. In North America, the vast majority of men have undergone circumcision. Only a Jew however, can have *brit milah*. Without the proper recitation of the associated blessings and the declaration by the parents that this procedure is being done so as to enter their son into an elevated relationship with God, the circumcision is merely a medical procedure.

"A sage should not live in a town without a *mohel*."

TALMUD BAVLI, SANHEDRIN 17B

કર્ય કર્ય કર્ય કર્ય કર્ય કર્ય કર્ય કર્ય કર્ય કર્ય કર્ય કર્ય કર્ય

Who performs a brit milah?

કર્ય કર્ય કર્ય કર્ય કર્ય કર્ય કર્ય કર્ય કર્ય કર્ય કર્ય કર્ય કર્ય

IN North America, *brit milah* is performed commonly in either of two ways. It may be done by a physician (Jewish, if possible) in conjunction with a rabbi or other Jew conversant with the ritual aspects of the ceremony. The more traditional, and in our view the far preferable choice, is to employ a *mohel*, often refered to in Yiddish as *"moyl"* or ritual circumciser.

In Biblical times, fathers usually circumcised their own sons, but by the common era, it became standard practice to employ a specialist to perform the *mitzvah* on one's behalf. To this day, the traditional practice is to begin the *brit milah* ceremony with a declaration by the father of his intention to carry out this *mitzvah* before the *mohel* or other person appointed by him actually does the procedure on his behalf.

Mohalim (plural of *mohel)* are usually rabbis and cantors who have undergone additional training in the specific medical procedure and religious laws pertaining to *brit milah*. Some received their training in the time-honored apprentice system, watching and assisting a master *mohel* (often their own fathers) perform hundreds of such procedures before going on their own. More often in modern times, a *mohel* (your grandma would say "*moyl,*" using the Yiddish word), has been trained in a major urban teaching hospital under the guidance of both rabbis and urologists. Most *mohalim* are Orthodox, though a fair number of Conservative and other non-Orthodox rabbis have this training, often from hospital programs in Israel.

Curiously, the physicians who are most comfortable in performing circumcisions are not, as one might think, urologists or pediatricians but rather obstetricians. This is because in hospitals where male babies are routinely circumcised unless the parents have made a specific request to the contrary, the procedure is done by the baby's mother's doctor—her obstetrician.

Why do we favor using a *mohel* over a physician/rabbi team? Our first son was born while we lived in New York; a locale with no shortage of *mohalim*. Though the bris (Ashkenazi Hebrew or Yiddish for *brit milah*) was on Saturday when travel is forbidden, our *mohel* had a network of homes at which he could stay so as to be present for us on *Shabbat*. We were nervous wrecks! After all the months of waiting, and the very difficult labor by which our first child came into the world, neither of us was all that eager to expose him to what seemed like so cruel a procedure.

All we remember is this: the blessing was said and the next thing we knew—it was literally a matter of seconds—our son was handed back to us for nursing and cuddling. No clamps. No long ordeal. A man who had performed truly countless circumcisions, our *mohel* was indeed a super-specialist. Several physician friends in attendance were utterly awe-struck at the amazing dexterity and technique the *mohel* displayed.

Our second son (and third child) was born eight days before Purim, in a city where there were no *mohalim*. We had little choice but to employ a Jewish doctor to do the actual procedure. Though the end result was fine, the procedure was more uncomfortable for the baby and took a much longer time to perform.

Dozens of *brit milah* ceremonies later, watching both physicians and *mohalim,* we have little doubt you'll thank yourself for choosing a *mohel.* That said, here are a few things to consider:

> Physician or *mohel,* reputation is everything. Ask your rabbi. Rabbis attend many such ceremonies each year. They know who is quick, competent and a *mensch.* This is not a service to choose from the Yellow Pages!

> Some physicians have special training in *brit milah.* The Reform movement has such a program in place in a few major cities. Again, your rabbi is the most trustworthy source of information in locating such a person.

> If you use a *mohel* who is Orthodox, and your rabbi is not, find out if the *mohel* is willing to participate with your rabbi. Some will not co-operate with non-Orthodox rabbis, though many will.

If you live in Rapid City, South Dakota (Jewish population approximately 20) or some other place where there is neither a *mohel* or Jewish physician, there are alternatives. Under such circumstances Halacha permits a non-Jew to do the actual cutting, as long as it is a Jew who conducts the ritual aspects (saying the blessings, naming the child, etc.). When possible, however, a Jewish circumcisor should be used.

You want the best for your baby. So too does the Royal Family of England, who surely can afford the best. Males of the English Monarchy are all circumcised, and in a country full of superb physicians, it has been long-standing tradition that the kings and princes of Great Britain are attended by none other than the Jewish Snowman family of London. Does your "prince" deserve less?

"Elijah traverses the universe, zealous to be present at every circumcision on the eighth day . . ."

ZOHAR 13A

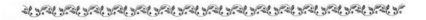

Why on the eighth day?

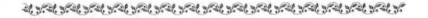

JEWS often seem to disagree on just about everything, from the politics of the middle east to basic theology. What question could one ask a member of an egalitarian *havurah* in Boston, a Yemenite Jew in Israel and the Lubavitcher Rebbe in Brooklyn and expect to receive the same answer?

Question: When does *brit milah* take place?

Answer: On the eighth day of the boy's life.

Amazing! Such unanimity! Unless there is a crucial medical reason in an individual case (such as very low birth weight), *brit milah* is always performed on the eighth day, following the instructions in the Torah: "At the age of eight days every male among you throughout the generations shall be circumcised." (*Genesis. 17:12* and repeated in *Leviticus 12:3*). This has been our practice since we received Torah, and there has never been a good reason to change it.

So important is the custom, that a *brit milah* may—indeed, must—be held on Yom Kippur if that is the child's eighth day of life. The *Schulchan Aruch* (the most widely known legal code) specifies that if one is a *mohel* one may even ignore certain of the laws of mourning, even for one's father or mother, in order to attend a *brit milah*.

What if the baby is born five days earlier than expected, and grandma and grandpa already purchased their non-refundable discount airline tickets and won't be able to come until the baby is 13 days old? But my sister's college graduation five hundred miles from here is scheduled for that very day! Why was my child born eight days before Superbowl Sunday?

Judaism is not always the most convenient religion. (Would it not be easier if all our holidays could come on Sundays, so we would not need to miss school or work?). We hold *brit milah* on the eighth day, as early as possible in the morning, not out of convenience, but for the same reason Abraham and Sarah did. *Brit milah* is the most tangible physical sign of our binding ourselves to God.

"Before honor goes humility."

PROVERBS 15:33

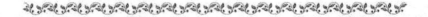

Do Jews have "godparents"?

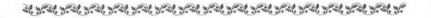

AT the *brit milah* ceremony for boys, it is customary to appoint a *kvater* (a man) and a *kvarterin* (a woman) whose ritual role is to bring the child into the room for the circumcision. In this manner, the *kvater* and *kvarterin* are honored at the *brit milah*. These people fill the role of "godparents" in Judaism.

Towards the end of the ceremony, all assembled pray together that the child will enter a life of "Torah, marriage and good deeds." In case of the death or incapacity of both parents, the *kvaterim* (plural, including both godfather and godmother), are charged with the responsibility to see that the child enters a life of Torah, marriage and good deeds. At the ceremony, therefore, you are publicly appointing the moral guardians of your child. In this light, the birth of children certainly calls for an update of one's legal will, even if you have few financial assets. For only via a legally drawn will can you be assured of the guardianship of your children, should both parents die while they are minors.

In addition to the *kvaterim,* who are responsible for nurturing, educating, and morally guiding a child in case they are needed, it is also traditional to appoint a *sandak.* The best translation of this word, is "man holding the baby while it is being circumcised." Sometimes the word is also translated as "godfather", but this fails to convey the true meaning.

The *sandak* is most often the boy's paternal grandfather, or a great-grandfather. Some families have the paternal grandfather act as *sandak* for one child's *bris,* and the maternal grandfather at a second or third child's *bris.* While there are no hard and fast rules, no one should serve as a *sandak* more than once.

The role of the *sandak,* other than to hold the baby at the ceremony, is to act as an elder, a sage, a voice of wisdom born of years. It is a great honor to be appointed as *sandak.*

The roles assigned to "godparents" are more than honorific. Talk to your brothers, sisters or friends before springing this decision upon them. Are they truly the kind of people you can fully trust with Jewishly educating and raising your child? To be true to the essence of Judaism, the decision of who to appoint to these roles should be made with deliberation, introspection, honesty and a bit of prayer.

"Behold how gladsome is circumcision that not
even the Sabbath defers it."

NEDARIM 31B

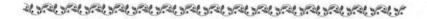

How should we prepare for the brit?

FIRST and foremost, you need
to have on hand whatever your doctor or *mohel* recommends
for care of the small wound created by the circumcision itself.
This usually consists of some sterile gauze pads and an
antiseptic ointment.

The *mohel* may examine the baby a few days before the *brit
milah* takes place to ascertain that the baby is large and healthy
enough to undergo the procedure. In addition, he will provide
a list of ritual and medical items needed for the ceremony. This
visit will give you the opportunity to ask questions and alleviate
some of the natural anxiety we all feel, particularly with our first
sons.

If your baby is given a pacifier, or if you bottle-feed, make
sure to have one on hand, as sucking gives infants a great sense
of comfort. Mothers who breast-feed will want to time feedings
that day so that the baby will be able to nurse immediately after
the *brit milah*.

The following is a list of required ritual items:

1. A place for the circumcision to take place, (a very stable table).
2. A pillow or cushion for the baby to lie on.
3. A chair to be left empty which will be designated during the ceremony as "the chair of Elijah."
4. A *tallit.* Some drape the *tallit* over Elijah's chair; others place the baby on it.
5. A *kiddush* cup with wine. Sweet, kosher wine is traditional. Your baby will be drinking a drop or two of it, so old-fashioned sweet wine is best. (If any of the major participants is an alcoholic, it is perfectly acceptable to use *kosher* grape juice instead.)
6. Photocopies of any responsive readings or prayers you wish guests to recite.
7. If you hold a traditional *seudat-mitzvah* (a full meal) afterwards, you may want to provide copies of *birkat hamazon* (the blessing after the meal, which has specific additions for the *brit milah*).
8. A hallah.

One thing you *don't* need for the *brit milah* is printed invitations. Since a *brit milah,* when done on the proper day, comes so soon after the birth, there is little time to send written invitations.

By tradition, it is considered such an important *mitzvah* to attend a *brit milah,* that the custom is to simply tell guests, "The *bris* will be Thursday at 10 o'clock at our house". In our own experience, we have found that we then had to explain to people the custom of not overtly inviting guests, and then adding the words, "we hope you can come."

Probably the most important preparation you need to do for the *brit* ceremony is psychological. If this is your first baby, you are experiencing a sudden loss of privacy and free-time now that this attention-demanding, twenty-four-hour-a-day visitor is making his home with you. Some people fear their first child's *bris* as overwhelming, and indeed it can feel that way. Part of the loveliness of our heritage as Jews is that the many friends and family who attend the *brit milah* help to diffuse the tension and anxiety we naturally feel.

Keep this in mind: babies circumcised in hospitals undergo the procedure alone, in a sterile, friendless environment, and afterwards cry themselves to sleep in solitary basinettes. Jewish babies are given wine to drink, are cuddled before, during and after the procedure, with their parents and dear ones feeling their discomfort with them. In a sense, the *brit milah* is a paradigm of all Jewish life, as we share each others pain and joy together as a community. Having a large circle of fellow Jews to rejoice and cry with you is bound to help.

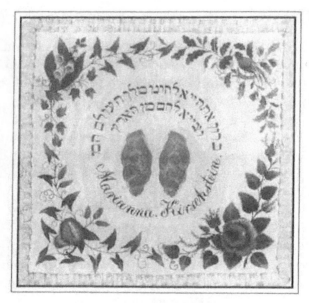

Embroidered Silk Hallah Cover
19th century Germany

"Abraham took Ishmael, his son, and all that were born in his house, and circumcised the flesh of their foreskin on the selfsame day."

GENESIS 17:23

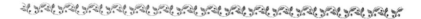

What is the structure of the brit milah *ceremony?*

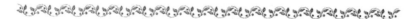

THE *brit milah* ritual is rather brief. Most often, it takes place at home. Though not essential, it is customary to have at least a *minyan* (a quorum of ten) on hand. Some parents find it more relaxing to hold the ceremony at a place other than their own home (e.g. synagogue or grandma's house).

A table is set aside for the procedure, with a pillow on it, and a chair is set aside which will be designated during the ceremony as *kisey shel Eliyahu*—"the chair of Elijah". (The prophet Elijah "visits" not only at the Passover *seder* but at all *brit milah* ceremonies as well.)

The *brit milah* ceremony begins when the baby boy is brought into the room by the *kvaterim*. All present stand and say, *"baruch ha-bah"* which means "Welcome! Blessed is he who is about to enter the covenant!" Frequently, the father or both parents may be called upon to read a prayer stating that this circumcision is specifically performed for the sake of entering their son into the covenant, and delegating to the *mohel* or physician the task of actually performing the *mitzvah*.

After the baby has been placed on the pillow, (or in traditional circles, on the lap of the *sandak*), the rabbi, *mohel or other officiant will usually explain the significance of the ceremony*, adding a *dvar torah* (literally "a word or two of Torah") to emphasize the religious nature of the gathering. The chair of Elijah is then designated, and his presence invoked. Sometimes the infant is placed on Elijah's chair for a moment before being returned to the place where the cirumcision will be performed.

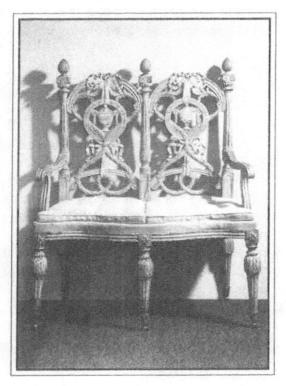

Carved Beechwood Circumcision Chair
Austria, 1791

At this point, *mohalim* and physicians who are in the practice of doing so will apply a clamp which draws back and holds the foreskin. This usually provokes the child to cry, often more than the incision itself. We have seen many *mohalim* do the procedure without any such clamps. Some will use topical anesthetics, though many Orthodox circumcisors will not do so on *halachic* (legal) grounds. There is debate on the matter.

With the *sandak* holding the baby so that he can not move, the officiant then pronounces the blessing: "We praise You, Eternal God for making our lives holy with *mitzvot*, and commanding us concerning circumcision". The circumcision is then performed; the procedure itself takes just a few seconds. After the circumcision is completed, the father (or in some places both parents) recite a blessing praising God, "for having bidden us enter our son into the covenant of Abraham our father".

At this point, all present say, *"keshem shenichnas labrit, ken yikanes l'torah, u'lechupah, u'lem'asim tovim*—As he has entered the covenant, so too may he enter a life of Torah, marriage and good deeds".

The officiant then recites a long blessing over a cup of wine, which includes a formal naming of the baby and a petition that he may grow to learn the full meaning of the covenant into which he has been brought. It is traditional to dip a finger or bit of gauze into the wine to give the baby some to drink. (Some even do so during the circumcision, to help calm the baby). Often, the rabbi or *mohel* will take a moment to explain the meaning of the baby's Hebrew name and if he is being named after a certain person. If the baby was not born to a halachically Jewish mother, many rabbis or *mohalim* will take the opportunity to recite a formula overtly stating that this is done *l'shem gerut*, that is, "for the sake of conversion." By doing so, along with a later visit to the *mikveh* the child's identity as a Jew will be acceptable to all streams of Judaism.

At the conclusion of the ceremony, special prayers are said on behalf of the infant. The traditional blessing is recited, "May God bless you and keep you. May God smile upon you and be gracious to you. May God look well upon you and grant you *shalom* (peace, or better "wholeness"). Sometimes, a few additional Psalms are added. In traditional circles, when a *minyan* is present, the entire assembly recites the *Alenu* prayer.

Of all life-cycle events, differences in customs of the various streams of Judaism are minimal concerning circumcision. By and large, *brit milah* is psychodynamically highly charged to begin with, and most people find adding very much to the ancient rite superfluous and artificial. It is precisely at moments such as these that the reassurance we feel in conducting ourselves in time-hallowed ways is strongest.

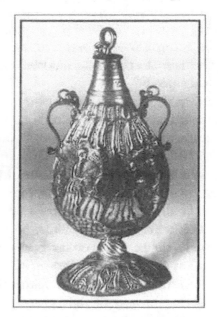

Silver Circumcision Powder Flask
18th century Moravia

"This is the day which the Lord has made; let us
rejoice and be glad therein."

PSALM 118:24

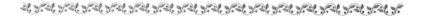

What sort of party should we plan?

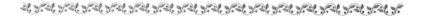

THE festive meal after any happy
life-cycle event is called *seudat mitzvah*.

There is great latitude in planning a *seudat mitzvah*. When
planning the menu, consider *kashrut* so that all the guests, both
observant and not, can enjoy the meal. Smoked fish such as lox,
creamed herring, whitefish, salads and the like are popular.
Nahit, (cold, salted chickpeas) are also common at a brit, as
well as alcoholic beverages. It is customary for guests to offer a
"l'chayim!". (a toast, "to life!"). Lifting a *shnapps* or two at a
bris, has been a healthy manifestation of the Jewish propensity
toward moderation in all things. As Ecclesiasties tells us, "To
every thing there is a season." That said, special care should still
be taken to make sure that non-alcoholic beverages are
available for guests with medical or chemical dependency
problems. Proper hospitality these days means thinking ahead
and providing for such special needs.

One of the traditional aspects of a *brit milah* is that, at the
conclusion of the festivities, a special version of *birkat
hamazon* (blessing after the meal) is recited. Some people

purchase or borrow special *benchers* (pamphlets with the special prayers printed inside) for the occasion. The traditional *halacha* is that one only recites the *birkat hamazon* after a meal that includes bread, and would therefore begin with the *motzi* blessing. If it is not your custom to recite *birkat hamazon,* it is still perfectly natural to begin the festivities with *ha-motzi* over hallah.

One of the blessings in the *birkat hamazon* refers to "shulchan zeh sh'achalnu alav" or, "this table, upon which we have eaten." Traditionally, this has been taken to mean that the festive meal is a full-scale sit-down affair. And, indeed, many people find, that after they include all the proper friends and relatives, they have a full scale celebration on their hands. This need not happen. A baby party can be lovely even when kept simple. Keep in mind that your guests are not expecting to attend a wedding or Bar Mitzvah! In our experience, simplicity has reinforced the real message that the party should convey, that this is a *seudat mitzvah*. Keep in mind that your table, even if you are serving a simple buffet, is like the altar in the sanctuary, and with that sentiment everything else will fall into place. Families are encouraged to share their good fortune with others in need through an act of tzedakah.

> "Forego not an occasion to observe a religious precept."
> TALMUD BAVLI, YOMA 33A

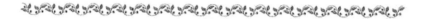

If we don't circumcise our baby, is he still a Jew?

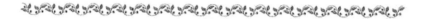

ACCORDING to traditional Jewish law (halacha), a baby born to a Jewish mother is considered a Jew whether or not he is circumcised. Failure of the parents to perform the *mitzvah* of *brit milah* does not alter the child's identity as a Jew.

Reform and Reconstructionist Judaism affirm "Patrilineal Descent." Children are extended a presumption of Jewish identity if either mother *or* father is a Jew when a declaration is made that the child is to be raised unambiguously as a Jew. A child's identity is affirmed by the timely performance of the customary life-cycle *mitzvot,* of which, for a male, *brit milah* is primary.

Traditionally, an uncircumcised male (called an *arel*) is considered a Jew, but such men are often not extended certain ritual honors, such as being called to the Torah or to lead the congregation in prayer. Rabbinic literature is rather complex on this matter, with some authorities denying the right of *sheva brachot* (the seven benedictions) to an uncircumcised groom, though none deny such a man the right to a Jewish wedding per se. Opinions in this century, even among some major Reform authorities, have upheld the correctness of maintaining such distinctions.

Brit milah is a unique *mitzvah*. Unlike the many *mitzvot* we choose for ourselves, no one asks an eight day old infant his opinion on the matter. The commandment is incumbant on the father, and failure to arrange for the timely entry of one's son into the covenant is universally seen as shirking a basic responsibility. If the father does not, then the mother ought to see to the *brit milah* herself. In *Exodus 4:24-26* we read a rather cryptic, enigmatic tale. Moses, for a reason we do not know, has neglected to circumcise his son and his wife Zipporah takes matters into her own hands. She *personally* performs the act (at the time done with a flint knife) and flings the foreskin at Moses, chastising him bitterly.

At various times in Jewish history, there were periods in which circumcision was neglected. The Bible describes how the generation which had wandered in the desert had not been circumcised; thus—before setting out into the promised land—all the males circumcised themselves in a mass act of community purification. (*Joshua 5:2-9*) Later, in the period of Greek cultural influence in Israel, some Jewish men even sought to "reverse" their circumcisions through painful building up of scar tissue (the plastic surgery of their day) so as to be more at home in the gymnasia.

In periods of severe persecution, especially during the Inquisition in Spain and the Holocaust in Europe, many Jewish parents sought to shield their sons from being known as Jews by witholding *brit milah*. Almost all modern rabbis have, at one time or another, needed to counsel men born in the Soviet Union or eastern European countries after World War II, who were not circumcised at birth for fear of another Holocaust.

Parents unswayed by arguments for circumcision from tradition ought at least keep these questions in mind:

> If the father *is* circumcised, what will the psychological impact be when the son recognizes that he is substantially *different* from his own father?

> What would happen if your son grows up to be religiously more traditional than his parents? *Halacha* (traditional Jewish law) is clear: once past the age of 13, the *mitzvah* becomes incumbant upon the son himself. Circumcision later in life is a far more serious and painful than the simple, relatively easy procedure done on the eighth day of life.

> What would be the son's feelings when, in summer camp or other situations where children see one another naked, he discovers that he is quite unlike all the other Jewish boys he knows? How can he grow up to feel like a Jew if he lacks this basic mark of the covenant?

A decision not to circumcise one's son, though not affecting his status as a Jew, may pose social problems for him later in life as circumcision is such a revered universal practice among Jews. Such a decision ought not to be made lightly.

"Many women have done excellently,
but you have surpassed them all."

PSALMS 31:29

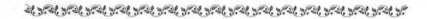

What kind of ceremony should we have for our daughter?

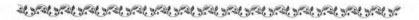

UNTIL the modern era, it was considered a great disability to be born female. Women were in little control of their own lives, had little control over property, had few ritual honors in houses of worship, and had little access to political power. No wonder the traditional *siddur* calls for men to recite a blessing every morning that praises God . . . "for not having made me a woman." Women—in seeming resignation to the Divine will—simply recite, "Praise be God, who has made me what I am."

Because daughters were seen as financial liabilities there was, for most of Jewish history, much more subdued rejoicing at the birth of a girl. Daughters, unlike sons, would not perpetuate family names and would not have the economic earning capacity as adults to support elderly parents. No wonder then, that in Jewish, (and most non-Jewish) traditions, pre-modern societies were much less jubilant concerning the birth of girls. To this day, the birth of a daughter is often simply marked by the father being called to the Torah on the *Shabbat* after the birth. A special prayer may be recited on the daughter's behalf, and her Jewish name announced to the community. The family may sponsor a *kiddush*, for the congregation. By and large, that was universal Jewish custom until the modern era.

"Classical" Reform Judaism distinguished itself a century ago by recognizing the birth of daughters as significant events. The Reform custom was, and still is in many locales, to call both parents to the *bimah* on a Friday evening soon after the birth of a baby (boy or girl), and to invoke God's blessings on the child and her parents. A formal naming would then take place followed by the presentation of a certificate. In many Reform, Conservative and Reconstructionist congregations these days, it is customary to bring the baby girl into the synagogue for a similar ceremony, at the end of which the rabbi might pronounce the traditional priestly blessing (the same one recited at the *brit* for boys).

In an effort to mark fully the complete equality of boys and girls in our era, many non-Orthodox families conduct a ceremony closely related to the *brit milah* ceremony for boys, adapted of course for girls. In addition to the more conventional "Naming Ceremony," the New Union Home Prayerbook (Reform) includes a "Covenant of Life" ceremony for girls, to be conducted in the home on the eighth day of life. The recently printed *Rabbi's Manual* (also Reform) includes a ceremony called *"hachnasat bat labrit*—Covenant Service For A Daughter," that even more closely parallels the *brit milah* ceremony. The Reconstructionist movement offers a *Brit Bnot Yisrael* ritual performed in the synagogue on Shabbat morning or at home on Saturday afternoon.

At present, there are literally dozens of highly personalized ceremonies circulating within the non-Orthodox community. Here are some elements you might include if you design your own ceremony:

1. Lighting candles, with or without an innovative blessing, perhaps "We Praise You Adonai, Eternal God, for enriching our lives with *mitzvot* and causing us to enter our daughter into the covenant of the Jewish people."
2. Appointing a chair for Elijah.
3. Appointing *kvaterim* (godparents) in the same manner as with boys.
4. Some people, in an attempt to make the ceremony as analogous as possible to *brit milah*, search for some tactile act to perform at this moment. You might consider these:

    Have the officiant wash the baby girl's feet, recalling the Biblical custom of foot-washing as a sign of hospitality and welcome. In this way, a *sandak* can also be involved.

    Have the officiant rub a small amount of olive oil on your daughter's forehead, recalling the Biblical image of annointing.

    Have the officiant wrap your baby in a *tallit*.

    Have the officiant physically place on object of Jewish significance into your daughter's hand, signifying in a ritual manner her capacity to perform *mitzvot*. This might be a Bible or a candlestick which you hope one day she may use to light Shabbat candles.
5. Include a formal naming at which your daughter's Hebrew name is announced and the significance explained. Some people also follow the custom of making an acrostic of the name using *Psalm 119* (each verse begins with a different Hebrew letter in alphabetical order). If you are capable or know someone who does Hebrew calligraphy, this can be a splendid concrete reminder of the day.

6. Include a *kiddush* over wine adding *shehechiyanu*, the blessing for happy occasions. He who recites the blessings drinks first, then shares the wine with the newborn and her parents.

Most rabbis are quite willing and even eager to help you design a creative, original ritual for your own daughter, or to officiate using one of the new standard liturgies. Be sure to discuss this matter with your rabbi. Home-based celebrations for girls can provide an opportunity for your own Jewish learning and commitment to grow. Take it as the pleasant, creative challenge it can be, and your *simhat-habat* (rejoicing over a new daughter), can be a wonderful and memorable occasion.

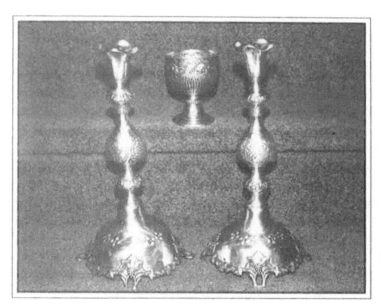

Traditional Shabbat Candlesticks and Cup
Stephen Wise Free Synagogue

> "For everything there is a season and a time
> for every purpose under heaven."
>
> ECCLESIASTES 3:1

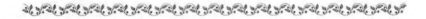

When should we have the ceremony for our daughter?

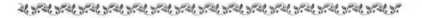

SIMHAT *habat, hachnasat bat labrit,* and other neologisms for the ceremonies modern Jews have created to welcome their daughters into the covenant have this in common: since they are not required by traditional *halacha,* there is great flexibility in when they can be held. They are not, traditionally, a *mitzvah she'hazman gramah,* "a commandment for which the time of performance is fixed." Some of the available liturgies are specifically worded to refer to the eighth day. Care should be taken when discussing your plans with your rabbi so that the appropriate liturgy will be used.

Many people feel rather strongly that such ceremonies for girls should be timed in the same manner as for a *brit milah* for boys, to stress the equality of the sexes. This may mean holding the ceremony on Shabbat or holidays, (if that is the eighth day of a girl's life). Keep in mind that there is leeway here. *Brit milah* takes precedence over any other scheduled event or activity. Since there are no such traditional strictures concerning ceremonies for girls, greater latitude might be extended in setting a time and place for the ceremony.

One possibility is to follow the paradigm suggested by *pidyon ha-ben* for firstborn sons. That ritual takes place any time after the thirtieth day of life, and concern for Shabbat and other family members' schedules are legitimate reasons for a slight delay. You might also find that, a full month after your daughter's birth, you will have more energy to plan a celebration at a more leisurely pace.

Whatever route you choose, the celebration for your new daughter ought not to be unduly delayed; it ought to be done when your daughter is still a young infant. In keeping with the sentiment of *brit milah* for boys, we do not ask our children if they want to enter the covenant; we make this decision for them. With effort and a bit of *mazal,* your children will affirm your decision at *Bar* or *Bat Mitzvah,* at Confirmation, later in life, but the initial act of entering the covenant is a duty incumbant not on the child but on the parent.

"Where a rule is uncertain in court and you are doubtful
of its virtue, follow the popular custom."

TALMUD YERUSHALMI, PEAH 7,5

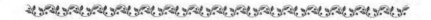

Can a boy have a naming ceremony?

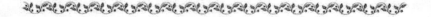

AN important aspect of both the
brit milah and the naming ceremony is the introduction of a
new, little person into the community. Traditionally a boy is
named at the *brit milah* ceremony on the eighth day of the
baby's life.

Each community has its own customs and standards as to
what is the correct and appropriate thing to do when naming a
baby. Some Reform, Conservative and Reconstuctionist
congregations offer naming ceremonies for both boys and girls.

The Law Committee of the Rabbinical Assembly, (the
professional organization of Conservative rabbis) has strongly
recommended that naming ceremonies for boys should not
take place, and that Conservative rabbis should not officiate at
them. It is necessary to check with your rabbi for the standards
and customs of your community.

> "A ceremony is not adequately discharged unless it is performed with beauty and dignity."
>
> M. H. LUZZATTO, MESILLAT YESHARIM

Who should perform the naming ceremony?

IF you belong to a synagogue, the proper person to officiate at any life cycle event is your rabbi. In larger congregations, the *hazzan* (cantor) often performs many of these duties. If you live in a Jewishly isolated community, or your synagogue does not have the services of a full-time rabbi or cantor, it is proper for any knowledgable Jewish adult to perform the ceremony. Parents should take an active role in bringing their children into the covenant. Rabbis' manuals are published by all the various streams in modern Judaism, and any Hebrew literate Jewish adult, with some preparation, can learn to officiate at a naming ceremony. Normally, the rabbi or cantor officiates because he or she is both the most knowledgable Jew in the community *and* an official representative of the community which the infant is about to join. In the absence of a rabbi or cantor, there is nothing wrong with having a "layperson" perform the ceremony, even if it means doing it yourself.

"Who are honorable? Those who honor others."

AVOT 4, 1

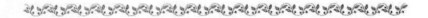

What honors are assigned at
a naming ceremony?

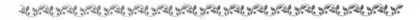

EVERY synagogue has its own local *minhagim* (customs). When naming ceremonies are conducted in the synagogue, most congregations limit the number of people who are to be called to the *bimah*. Naming ceremonies that take place on Friday evenings in a Temple normally include only the parents and sometimes the baby, although some permit the inclusion of godparents.

In congregations where the traditional number of *aliyot* are called to the Torah on a Saturday morning, there are more opportunities to honor family members. A minimum of seven people are given the honor of reciting the blessings over the Torah reading, other people are called to dress and lift the Torah. In congregations where this is not the practice, godparents and grandparents might be given the honor of opening or closing the ark at the appropriate moments, or lighting Shabbat candles or reciting a prayer of thanksgiving.

Home ceremonies have more latitude. People you wish to honor might have the role of holding the baby, carrying her into the room, reciting one or more of the blessings, especially *ha-motzi* at the start of the festive meal.

Again, the important thing to keep in mind is that the role of *kvaterim* (godparents) should be assigned thoughtfully, with full cognizance of the position.

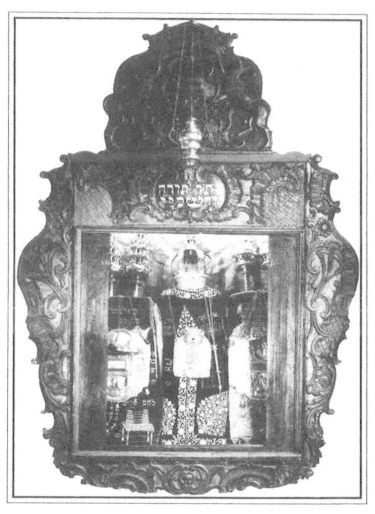

Torah Ark
Masbach Germany, 1760

"A good name is better than great riches."

PROVERBS 22:1

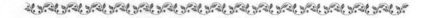

Does the baby receive a certificate?

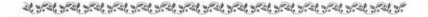

ALTHOUGH some Orthodox *mohalim* do not issue a certificate of *brit milah,* majority practice in North America is that boys receive such a certificate at their *brit milah.* Girls receive a certificate at their naming or other celebration marking their entrance into the covenant. Each of the streams have printed, standard certificates, some of which are quite beautiful. Your synagogue office carries a stock of such items. Many Jewish bookstores also carry such supplies. (If you live in relative Jewish isolation, most stores are quite willing to conduct transactions by mail.)

The certificate contains a place for the baby's full English and Hebrew name. Don't lose the certificate! When your child begins religious school, you will need to know his or her Hebrew name. For *Bar/Bat Mitzvah,* Confirmation and for their weddings (the *ketubah* or wedding contract requires the full Hebrew names of the bride and groom), the certificate your child receives as an infant will be the authoritative document. Keep it in a safe place.

"A convert is regarded as an infant, newborn."

TALMUD BAVLI, YEVAMOT 22A

Can a baby convert to Judaism?

USUALLY, conversion to Judaism requires consent, but when it comes to small children, the rabbis made an exception. They ruled that the parents are allowed to make that decision for the child, reasoning that conversion is an act that is done for the child's benefit. It can, therefore, be performed early in life. Later, if the child wishes to renounce Jewish status, that can be done at the age of majority. (Some consider this to be the age of *Bar/Bat Mitzvah*, when Jewish children are expected to take on the responsibilities of our faith.)

The answer to the question of who is and who is not a Jew varies, depending upon whom you ask. In Orthodox and Conservative circles, a baby must be born of a Jewish mother. In Reform and Reconstructionist circles, a child may be considered a Jew if one parent, (it doesn't matter which), is a Jew, and if the child is being raised exclusively as a Jew. If the parents wish the child to be recognized unambiguously as Jewish by all members of the community, this can easily be accomplished by ritual conversion early in the child's life.

For a male, this can be partially accomplished at the *brit milah* on the eighth day of the child's life. The *mohel,* or rabbi recites the appropriate extra prayers and blessings for the conversion during the *brit* ceremony. The conversion is not complete, however, until the baby is taken to the *mikveh,* (ritual bath) and, therefore, the child's Hebrew name is not formally bestowed upon him during the brit ceremony. A *mikveh* is a warm pool, a portion of which must be rainwater, built in a ritually prescribed manner. A parent enters the *mikveh* holding the baby, and participates in the entire event with the child. The baby is fully immersed in the water for a moment, in the same manner as might be done at an infant swim class. After the immersion in the *mikveh,* the child receives his Hebrew name, and is considered to be halachically Jewish by all standards. Usually, a certificate attesting to the child's new status is issued at that time.

It is necessary for the circumcision to heal before the baby can be fully immersed in water. This fact separates the *brit milah* and the ritual immersion by a short period of time. This should be determined by your doctor or *mohel.*

Sometimes it occurs that a boy is circumcised medically at birth, and later wishes to become Jewish. If this is the case, a ceremony called *"hatafat dam brit"* is performed in conjuction with *mikveh,* where one drop of blood is ritually and painlessly drawn from the glans of the penis. Some Reform and Reconstructionist rabbis do not insist upon it.

Girls are also taken to the *mikveh* for ritual immersion, and may then receive their Hebrew names. After this event, a naming ceremony may be performed for public recognition of the child's entrance into the covenant. Girls also receive a special certificate attesting to their new status.

For further information concerning conversion, *mikveh,* and the nature of the procedure, your rabbi should be consulted.

"The Lord to spoke to Moses saying: Consecrate
to Me every firstborn, man and beast, the first issue
of every womb among the Israelites is Mine."

EXODUS 13:1-2

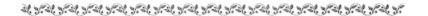

What is pidyon ha-ben?

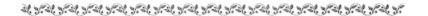

JUDAISM has ancient roots. Jews
have kept various customs and traditions alive over the course
of the millennia, and of all the rituals we maintain and observe,
pidyon ha-ben, the act of redeeming a firstborn son, truly
smacks of antiquity.

In ancient days, it was commonly believed that the gods were
entitled to the first fruits and vegetables of both field and
womb. The first fruits at harvest time, firstborn animals, and
firstborn humans, were all ritually sacrificed to the gods.

Judaism left these primitive rites behind, and instead
substituted a new custom. Any firstborn male, the "first issue"
of a woman's womb, (known in Hebrew as *peter rechem*,) was
to be consecrated to God as a priest, or as a religious
representative in the local communities of the time. This didn't
last long, however, for, as the story goes, God changed His mind
after the golden calf episode at Mount Sinai. When God saw the
firstborn males committing idolatry, He offered the priestly
responsibilities to the Levites, who then became God's ritual

helpers on earth. Since that time, we follow the custom of releasing the firstborn male child of his ancient obligation with the following ceremony.

A table is set with a hallah and a kiddush cup. The mother brings in the baby and hands him to the father who is facing a Kohen, a Jew who traces his ancestry to the priestly class. The father has obtained five pieces of silver, (silver dollars are often used), and has a dialogue with the *Kohen*.

The *Kohen* asks the father if he wishes to surrender his son for priestly service, or if he wishes to ransom him for five pieces of silver. The father replies that he prefers to keep his son. (No other answer is acceptable). He then recites two blessings and gives the *Kohen* the silver coins. Then the *Kohen* recites three times, "Your son is redeemed. Your son is redeemed. Your son is redeemed." A blessing is said over the hallah and the wine, and a festive meal is served to the invited guests. The ceremony is known as *pidyon ha-ben,* literally meaning the redemption of the son.

This ceremony may take place any time after the thirtieth day of life, whether there has been a *brit milah* or not. (Sometimes a brit is postponed due to the ill health of the baby.) Thirty days is the age at which a baby is considered to be halachically viable. *Pidyon ha-ben* may not take place on Shabbat or holidays where there are prohibitions against spending money.

This ritual need only be performed if the child is a male, the first "issue" of the womb, and if the father is not a *Kohen* or *Levite*. These rules exclude babies born of cesarean section, (for the baby is not considered to have "issued forth"), and babies born after a previous miscarriage. Each woman can have only one firstborn, not one per husband, and if the firstborn is a girl, the law tells us that the ceremony does not take place.

Today, as we accord similar honors to both male and female children, some like to celebrate the ritual for girls as well. A *pidyon ha-bat* (redemption of the daughter ceremony), though a departure from the traditional halachah, can be seen as a warm expression of gratitude. In this case, no money need actually be exchanged, though a symbolic gift of *tzedakah* in the child's name would certainly be appropriate.

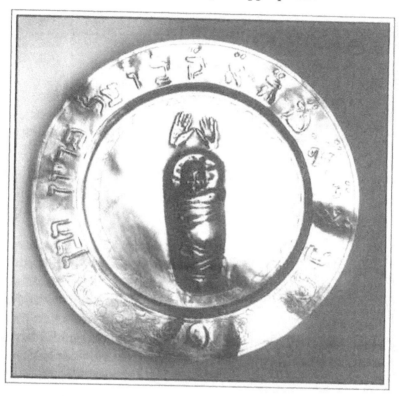

Brass Plate for Redemption of the First-Born
18th century Eastern Europe

"A happy heart gives life to man,
joyfulness lengthens his days."

BEN SIRA 30,12

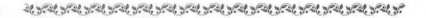

What is shalom zachor?

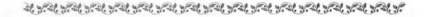

IT is customary in some communities to mark the first Shabbat of a male child's life with a special celebration. On that Friday night, after dinner, relatives and friends gather at the baby's home to congratulate the family.

Biblical passages and psalms are recited, and a *d'var Torah* might be given. A light meal is also served. In some places, lentils and chickpeas (nahit) are traditional foods because of their round shape, symbolizing life's continuity.

Shalom zachor literally means "greeting the male." In Arabic, the event is known as *shasha*, or *blada*.

As we now celebrate the birth of a female with the same joy as that of a male, some hold this gathering in honor of their baby girls as well. The only thing that needs to be changed is the name of the event. It becomes *"shalom nekevah,"* greeting the female, or *"shalom bat,"* greeting the daughter.

> "Memory is cottonwool that soaks up everything."
>
> MAIMONIDES, COMMENTARY ON MISHNAH AVOT

What is a wimpel?

IN western Europe, an interesting custom arose. The linen wrap worn by the baby at his *brit milah* was made into an embroidered Torah binder. The special piece of fine linen that was selected for the baby's swaddling cloth, was cut into stripes, six inches wide, and sewn together to form a long ribbon. On it, the mother would then embroider the baby's name, date of birth, astrological sign, and any wishes that she might have for her new baby. These included wishes for a life of Torah, *mitzvot*, good deeds, and a good marriage.

The finished wimpel was presented to the family's congregation after the baby's first birthday. A small ceremony accompanied the presentation. Usually, the child was carried to the *bimah* after the conclusion of the Torah service, where the rabbi would offer a blessing over him. Then the wimpel was publicly displayed, and used that day as the Torah binder.

Many synagogues kept these wimpels in their archives, where they served as an important part of the historical record of the congregation. Unfortunately, most of these wimpels were lost during World War II, and no longer exist.

This human interest story recently appeared in our local Jewish newspaper:

An older man, a survivor of the Holocaust recently toured an exhibit of memorabilia from Germany. Among the Torah scrolls, *yads*, and personal artifacts, was a selection of wimpels that had been rescued from a Nazi collection of Jewish relics. One of the pieces in that collection was the wimpel that had been made for him by his mother!

This custom of wimpel-making is enjoying a revival today, as more and more Jews seek to make old traditions meaningful once again. Making a wimpel for your new baby is one way to express your creativity in an authentic Jewish art form, as well as an opportunity to create a historic momento for your baby and for the Jewish community as a whole.

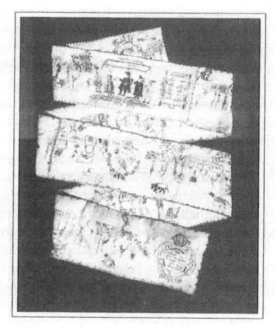

Wimpel
Germany, 1771

"What God is to the world, parents are to their children."

PHILO OF ALEXANDRIA, COMMENTARY TO DEUTERONOMY 14:1

What are parents' obligations to their children?

SOME people subscribe to a philosophy of parenting that sounds something like this: In order to raise happy and emotionally healthy children, you simply need to offer love and understanding. If you give them that, everything else will fall into place.

While it is true that love is a wonderful and important aspect of parenting, and that there is certainly no objection in Judaism to offering your child lots of love, our tradition does not stop there. With concern for the times when things might not always fall into place, all aspects of financial and custodial responsibility are expounded upon in the Talmud. Such issues as divorce, custody, educational duties, the age at which a child is no longer a dependent, are all discussed.

This Talmudic excerpt is often quoted. A parents' obligations are, "to circumcise him, to redeem him, to teach him Torah, to find him a wife, to teach him a trade," and some say, "to teach him to swim that he may save his life." If we look at this statement with modern eyes with all its implications, and then gender neutralize it, it becomes a fairly complete list of our modern expectations as well.

Today, as then, we still bring our children into the covenant, (with naming ceremonies and *brit milah*), we still spend great energy and expense on education, we still require that our children be trained in a profession from which they will gain both personal and financial reward, and we still attempt to teach our children to protect themselves from the hazards of life, whether that be by teaching them to swim or by some other means. We would still like to find our children appropriate spouses, though they don't often permit it.

Perhaps there is a stereotype of an overly doting Jewish parent, providing to excess. As with all stereotypes, there may be some truth to it. However, by offering our children more than just love, we follow the example of generations past, who did their utmost to provide their children with a secure and successful future.

"Train up a child in the way he should go, and even when he is old, he will not depart from it."

PROVERBS 22:6

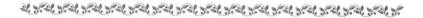

What role do children play in Jewish tradition?

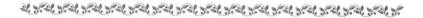

An ancient midrash follows:

When Moses was offered the Torah on Mount Sinai, God asked for collateral before giving something so precious. God asked Moses to approach the people for a proper symbol of the covenant. First, the Jews offered their jewelry, but God countered that the Torah was more precious than jewels. Next, Moses offered our great leaders as the sign, but God wouldn't accept this either, for God said that our leaders were already committed. Finally, after much thought, the Jewish people offered their children to God, promising to teach their children Torah throughout the generations. This, the most precious gift a human being can offer, was acceptable to God, and we have been diligently teaching our children Torah ever since. *(Song of Songs Rabah)*

During the recitation of the Shema, we repeat this same promise with the words: "You shall teach these words diligently onto your children." Our tradition has many vehicles with which we can accomplish this awesome task, only one of which is formal schooling. We teach by personal example, by observing the mitzvot, and by bringing Judaism and the Jewish holidays into our homes.

Almost every holiday has a special role for children to play, making children central to our celebrations. The Passover seder, for example, is designed as a learning experience for children. Complete with stories, symbols that you can eat, active participation, (opening the door for Elijah), and the specific role of the recitation of the Four Questions, Passover is a home holiday that invites the participation of children.

The same goes for Simhat Torah, Purim and Hanukkah. It is our children who create the noise and the enthusiasm, who play the holiday games with a passion to win. Even at the Shabbat table, we take the time to bless each child individually.

The Torah portion known as the "Binding of Isaac" tells of God's demand that Abraham sacrifice his only son, Isaac. It ends, however with the words, "and they rose up and went together to Beer-sheba." It is significant that after all the trials and tests to which God subjects Abraham and his son Isaac, they are able to walk on in life together, to remain forever bound by that invisible thread of faith. We too are inextricably bound to our children. They are our collateral, we are their teachers. We help them grow, and in return, they keep us vital and strong.

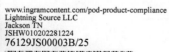